DIABETIC JUICING

COOKBOOK

80+ Fast and Easy Recipes to Immediately Detox your Body and regulate your Blood Sugar level | Easy-to-find Ingredients

TABLE OF CONTENTS

INTRODUCTION

The Diabetic Juicing Cookbook is a comprehensive guide designed to help diabetic people manage their condition through a healthy and balanced diet. This cookbook features a collection of delicious and nutritious juicing recipes tailored to meet the unique needs of people with diabetes. With a focus on delicious fresh fruits, vegetables, and other healthy ingredients, these recipes are designed to help regulate blood sugar levels, improve overall health, and provide essential vitamins and minerals. Whether you're new to juicing or are looking for new recipes to add to your routine, the Diabetic Juicing Cookbook has everything you need to start enjoying the many benefits of juicing for diabetes management.

WHY THIS BOOK?

The Diabetic Juicing Cookbook is a comprehensive guide for those looking to improve their nutrition, lose weight, and manage their diabetes through juicing. It offers a unique approach to managing diabetes by incorporating fresh, nutrient-rich juices into one's diet. The recipes included in the book are carefully crafted to meet the unique needs of people with diabetes, taking into consideration factors such as calorie count, carbohydrate content, and the glycemic index of ingredients.

The book covers all aspects of juicing for diabetes management, from the basics of juicing and the benefits of incorporating juices into your diet to a comprehensive list of ingredients, tips on selecting and storing produce, and recipes for all occasions. The delicious recipes in the book are designed to be easy to prepare, delicious, and nutritious, providing a convenient and tasty way to get the nutrients and fiber your body needs.

In addition to recipes, the book also includes helpful information and tips on managing diabetes, such as the importance of monitoring blood sugar levels, ways to reduce the risk of complications, and practical advice on meal planning. Whether you're new to juicing or are looking for new and healthy ways to manage your diabetes, the Diabetic Juicing Cookbook has everything you need to get started.

With its focus on healthy and balanced juicing, the Diabetic Juicing Cookbook is an essential resource for anyone looking to improve their health, manage their diabetes, and achieve their weight loss goals.

CHAPTER 1
UNDERSTANDING DIABETES

Diabetes is characterized by abnormally high amounts of blood glucose or blood sugar in the blood. The glucose in your bloodstream comes from the food you consume. Glucose is an essential source of fuel for the cells in your body. Insulin is a hormone that makes it easier for glucose to enter the body's cells. Insulin is responsible for this.

The inability of the body to manufacture insulin is one of the defining characteristics of type 1 diabetes. When you have diabetes, your body cannot create enough insulin or make good use of the insulin it produces. If you do not have an adequate amount of insulin in your body, glucose will build up in your blood, ultimately resulting in diabetes.

Foods that affect blood sugar levels

Certain foods, known as carbohydrates or "carbs," are the source of the sugar in your blood. Candies and other sweets, soft drinks, bread, tortillas, and white rice contain a high carbohydrate concentration. Your blood sugar level will rise directly to the number of carbohydrates you consume.

If you have diabetes of either type 1 or type 2, making smart decisions about the foods you eat is essential to maintaining appropriate blood sugar levels. If you can keep your blood sugar under control, you will minimize your risk of developing major health complications due to diabetes, such as loss of vision and issues with your heart.

Eating meals that maintain your blood sugar levels healthily will help prevent diabetes in the future, which is especially important if you have a history of diabetes or are at risk for having diabetes.

CHAPTER 2
NUMBER OF DIABETICS IN THE USA

Diabetes is a serious health issue that affects millions of people in the United States. As of 2021, it is estimated that over 34 million people in the country have been diagnosed with diabetes, which is nearly 10% of the total population. It is estimated that another 88 million people have prediabetes, which indicates a high risk of developing diabetes near future. This number continues to rise each year.

The ever-increasing incidence of diabetes in the United States demonstrates how critical it is to find effective treatments for this ailment. Diabetes is a chronic condition that badly affects how the body processes glucose (sugar). It is a leading cause of serious health complications, such as heart disease, stroke, renal disease, and blindness. The condition can also lead to amputations. It can be a substantial struggle for people with diabetes to maintain control of their blood sugar levels through appropriate eating, regular physical exercise, and careful administration of their medication.

The rising percentage of diabetes in the United States puts a strain on the country's healthcare infrastructure, with direct and indirect costs estimated to amount to hundreds of billions of dollars each year. This highlights the need for ongoing research and advances in diabetes care, as well as the importance of diabetes prevention and management efforts, including education and awareness, lifestyle changes, and access to care.

Overall, the growing number of people with diabetes in the United States highlights the need for increased focus and resources on diabetes prevention and management, as well as the ongoing impact of this condition on public health and the healthcare system.

Diet for diabetes

There must be some specific diets or meal plans adaptable to each individual's needs. Your primary care physician may recommend that you consult with a registered dietitian so that they can assist you in developing the optimal diet for you. The following will be taken into consideration by the plan:

- Any medications that you now use
- How much you weigh
- Any additional medical issues that you suffer from
- Your way of life and your preferences.
- Your aspirations

Eating the appropriate meals, in the appropriate amounts, at the appropriate times and appropriate interval is a component shared by all diabetes diet programs.

Foods I can eat

Consuming a wide variety of nutritious foods from each of the following food groups is essential for managing diabetes effectively through diet:

- Fruits and fresh vegetables
- Whole grains, including wheat, brown rice, barley, oats, and quinoa, are healthier than refined grains.
- Proteins, such as meat, chicken, turkeys, fish, eggs, nuts, fresh beans, lentils, and tofu
- Proteins, such as meat, chicken, fresh turkey, fish, and eggs
- Dairy products like milk, yogurt, and cheese are nonfat or low-fat.

Foods to avoid

You should consume fewer foods and beverages that are heavy in carbohydrates to maintain a healthy blood sugar level. This does not preclude the possibility that you will ever appreciate them. However, you will need to consume them less frequently or in lower quantities than usual.

Below are some foods to avoid:

- Candies, delicious cookies, cake, ice cream, cereals, and canned fruits with sugar are foods high in sugar.
- Juice, ordinary soda or soft drinks, and regular sports drinks are examples of beverages with added sugars.
- White Rice, tortillas, bread, and pasta should be avoided.
- Vegetables are high in starch, including white potatoes, corn, and peas.

You should reduce the amount of alcohol you consume and the amount of fat and salt in your diet.

Things to consider

If you have diabetes, you must consume the appropriate meals daily. Your eating plan will specify how much food you should consume at each meal and snack to consume the appropriate amount of carbohydrates. You will learn how to measure your food and count the carbohydrates in your food.

Consuming approximately the same number of carbohydrates at each meal can be beneficial.

You will also learn how to adhere to your eating plan when you are eating at home as well as when you are eating in a restaurant. Eating healthily to maintain control of your blood sugar levels requires some work. However, the reward is enjoying your life to the fullest while managing diabetes.

CHAPTER 3
BENEFITS OF USING A BALANCED DIET AND JUICES FOR DIABETICS

A proper, balanced, and healthy diet, along with daily fresh vegetable and fruit juices, can have several potential benefits for people with diabetes. Some of the key benefits include:

Better Blood Sugar Control: Consuming a diet rich in fresh fruits and vegetables and incorporating fresh juices into the diet can help improve blood sugar control by providing a steady source of nutrients and reducing the need for rapid insulin spikes.

Improved Nutrient Intake: Fresh juices can be a great way to increase nutrient intake, including vitamins, minerals, nutrients, and antioxidants, which are crucial for overall health and managing diabetes.

Weight Management: Incorporating fresh juices into a balanced diet can help with weight management by reducing calorie intake, providing a source of nutrient-dense, low-calorie beverages, and promoting feelings of fullness.

Improved Heart Health: Diabetes can cause heart disease, and a diet rich in fresh fruits and vegetables, along with fresh juices, can help improve heart health by reducing inflammation, reducing blood pressure, and improving cholesterol levels.

Improved Gut Health: Fresh juices can also help enhance gut health by promoting the growth of good bacteria and reducing inflammation, which can help improve overall health and manage diabetes.

Overall, incorporating fresh vegetable and fruit juices into a proper, balanced, and healthy diet can have several potential benefits for people with diabetes, including better blood sugar control, improved nutrient intake, weight management, heart health, and gut health.

Things to know about choosing fruits and vegetables

When choosing fruits and vegetables for juicing, there are several important factors to consider:

Variety: To get the most nutritional benefits, it is important to choose various fruits and vegetables. This will ensure you get a wide range of vitamins, minerals, and antioxidants.

Seasonality: Fruits and vegetables in season tend to be fresher and more nutrient-dense. Consider incorporating seasonal produce into your juicing regimen to get the most health benefits.

Quality: Choose high-quality fruits and vegetables free from bruises, mold, or other signs of damage. Select organic produce whenever possible to reduce exposure to pesticides and other harmful chemicals.

Glycemic Index: For people with diabetes, choosing fruits and vegetables with a low glycemic index is important, meaning they do not cause rapid spikes in blood sugar levels. Fruits such as berries and vegetables such as leafy greens are typically lower on the glycemic index.

Personal Preferences: Finally, choosing fruits and vegetables you enjoy is important to be more likely to follow your juicing regimen. Experiment with different combinations and find what works best for you.

By considering these factors when choosing fruits and vegetables for juicing, you can help ensure that you get the most nutritional benefits and effectively manage your diabetes.

CHAPTER 4
BEST VEGETABLES AND FRUITS FOR DIABETIC PATIENTS

For people with diabetes, choosing fruits and vegetables that are really low on the glycemic index and provide a steady source of nutrients and fiber is important. Some of the best options include:

Leafy greens: Spinach, kale, and lettuce are all low on GI and high in fiber and nutrients like vitamins A and C, iron, and calcium.

Berries: Berries such as strawberries, raspberries, and blueberries are low on the GI and high in fiber and antioxidants like anthocyanins and Vitamin C.

Cruciferous vegetables: Vegetables like broccoli, cauliflower, and Brussels sprouts are low in the GI and high in fiber, vitamins, and minerals. They are also a great source of specific antioxidants.

Tomatoes are low on the GI and rich in fiber, vitamin C, and potassium.

Citrus fruits: Oranges, lemons, and limes are high in fiber and Vitamin C.

Avocado: Avocados have less healthy monounsaturated fats and antioxidants.

Apples: Apples are low in GI and high in fiber and antioxidants.

Incorporating these fruits and vegetables into your juicing regimen can help regulate blood sugar levels, improve nutrient intake, and support overall health and wellness.

CHAPTER 5
JUICE RECIPES

Green Power: kale, spinach, cucumber, celery, green apple, lemon

Serving size: 1 cup (240 ml)

Servings per recipe: Approximately 1

Nutritional values per serving:

- Calories: 35
- Total fat: 0.3 g
- Saturated fat: 0 g
- Trans fat: 0 g
- Cholesterol: 0 mg
- Sodium: 53 mg
- Total Carbohydrate: 9 g
- Dietary Fiber: 2.2 g
- Sugars: 5 g
- Protein: 1.5 g

Ingredients:

- Two cup kale
- Two cup spinach
- One cucumber
- Two stalks of celery
- One green apple
- One lemon
- Two cups of liquid base

Instructions:

1. Wash and chop the kale, spinach, cucumber, celery, and green apple.
2. Squeeze the lemon to get the juice.
3. Add the chopped greens, cucumber, celery, green apple, lemon juice, and liquid base to a blender.
4. Add any optional ingredients if desired.
5. Blend until smooth, about 1-2 minutes, or until desired consistency is reached.
6. Pour into a glass and enjoy immediately.

This smoothie is made with vitamins, minerals, and antioxidants, making it a great choice for anyone looking to support a healthy lifestyle, especially those with diabetes. Enjoy!

Berry Blast: strawberries, blueberries, raspberries, blackberries, almond milk

Serving size: 1 cup (240 ml)

Servings per recipe: Approximately 1

Nutritional values per serving:

- Calories: 68
- Total fat: 2 g
- Saturated fat: 0 g
- Trans fat: 0 g
- Cholesterol: 0 mg
- Sodium: 93 mg
- Total Carbohydrate: 13 g
- Dietary Fiber: 4 g
- Sugars: 7 g
- Protein: 1.7 g

Ingredients:

- One cup or 236 grams of strawberries
- One cup or 236 grams of blueberries
- One cup or 236 grams of raspberries
- One cup or 236 grams of blackberries
- One cup or 236 grams of almond milk

Instructions:

1. Wash and chop the strawberries, blueberries, raspberries, and blackberries.
2. Add the mixed berries and almond milk to a blender.
3. Add any optional ingredients if desired.
4. Blend until smooth, about 1-2 minutes, or until desired consistency is reached.
5. Pour into a glass and enjoy immediately.

This smoothie is bursting with flavor and nutrition, thanks to its mix of fresh, juicy berries.

Carrot Orange: carrots, oranges, Ginger

Serving size: 1 cup (240 ml)

Servings per recipe: Approximately 1

Nutritional values per serving:

- Calories: 65
- Total Fat: 0.2 g
- Saturated Fat: 0 g
- Trans Fat: 0 g
- Cholesterol: 0 mg
- Sodium: 82 mg
- Total Carbohydrates: 16.4 g
- Dietary Fiber: 3 g
- Sugars: 3.3 g
- Protein: 1.3 g

Ingredients:

- Two cups carrots
- Two oranges
- One piece of Ginger
- One cup liquid base

Instructions:

1. Wash and chop the carrots, oranges, and Ginger.
2. Add the carrots, oranges, Ginger, and liquid base to a blender.
3. Add any optional ingredients if desired.
4. Blend until smooth, about 1-2 minutes, or until desired consistency is reached.
5. Pour into a glass and enjoy immediately.

This smoothie is made with vitamins, minerals, and antioxidants, thanks to its mix of fresh, juicy oranges and nutrient-rich carrots. The Ginger adds a zesty kick that complements the sweetness of the oranges and carrots. Enjoy!

Sweet Beet: beets, apples, Ginger

Serving size: 1 cup (240 ml)

Servings per recipe: Approximately 1

Nutritional Information per serving:

- Serving size: 1 cup (240 ml)
- Calories: 95
- Total Fat: 0.3g
- Saturated Fat: 0g
- Trans Fat: 0g
- Cholesterol: 0mg
- Sodium: 52mg
- Total Carbohydrates: 23.6g
- Dietary Fiber: 3.2g
- Sugars: 6.2g
- Protein: 1.5g

Ingredients:

- Two beets, peeled well

- Two apples

- One piece of Ginger

- One cup liquid base

Instructions:

1. Wash and chop the beets, apples, and Ginger.

2. Add the beets, apples, Ginger, and liquid base to a blender.

3. Add any optional ingredients if desired.

4. Blend until smooth, about 1-2 minutes, or until desired consistency is reached.

5. Pour into a glass and enjoy immediately.

This smoothie is made with vitamins, minerals, and antioxidants thanks to its mix of sweet, juicy apples and nutrient-rich beets. The Ginger adds a zesty kick that complements the sweetness of the beets and apples. Enjoy!

Citrus Sunrise: oranges, grapefruits, lemons, limes

Serving size: 1 cup (240 ml)

Servings per recipe: Approximately 2

Nutritional Information per serving:

- Calories: 148
- Total Fat: 0.6 grams
- Saturated Fat: 0.1 grams
- Cholesterol: 0 milligrams
- Sodium: 1 milligram
- Total Carbohydrates: 38 grams
- Dietary Fiber: 7.6 grams
- Total Sugars: 8 grams
- Protein: 3 grams

Ingredients:

- Four oranges, peeled and segmented

- Two grapefruits, peeled and segmented

- One lemon, juiced

- One lime, juiced

Instructions:

1. In a Juicer or blender, combine the orange and grapefruit segments.

2. Squeeze the lemon and lime juice into the blender and mix everything.

3. Serve immediately in glasses, garnished with a wedge of lemon or lime if desired.

Enjoy this refreshing and healthy diabetic-friendly recipe! The natural sweetness of citrus fruits provides a satisfying sweetness without adding sugars.

Melon Madness: watermelon, cantaloupe, honeydew, mint

Serving size: 1 cup (240 ml)

Servings per recipe: Approximately 2

Nutritional Information per serving:

- Calories: 47
- Total Fat: 0.3g
- Saturated Fat: 0g
- Trans Fat: 0g
- Cholesterol: 0mg
- Sodium: 26mg
- Total Carbohydrates: 12
- Dietary Fiber: 9g
- Sugars: 3g
- Protein: 5g

Ingredients:

- Four cups watermelon
- Four cups cantaloupe
- Four cups honeydew melon
- 1/4 cup chopped mint leaves

Instructions:

1. In a Juicer or blender, combine the watermelon, cantaloupe, and honeydew melon.

2. Gently mix in the chopped mint leaves.

3. Serve chilled in glasses, garnished with additional mint leaves if desired.

This Melon Madness recipe is a delicious and refreshing way to enjoy the natural sweetness of melons while keeping your blood sugar levels in check. The mint adds a cool and refreshing flavor that perfectly complements the melons' sweetness.

Cucumber Cooler: cucumber, lime, mint

Serving size: 1 cup (240 ml)

Servings per recipe: Approximately 2

Nutritional Information per serving:

- Calories: 12
- Total Fat: 0.1 grams
- Saturated Fat: 0 grams
- Cholesterol: 0 milligrams
- Sodium: 2 milligrams
- Total Carbohydrates: 3 grams
- Dietary Fiber: 1 gram
- Total Sugars: 1 gram
- Protein: 1 gram

Ingredients:

- Four large cucumbers, peeled and sliced
- Two limes juiced
- ½ cup chopped mint

Instructions:

1. Combine the sliced cucumbers, lime juice, and chopped mint leaves in a Juicer.
2. Blend until mixed well.
3. Pour into glasses and enjoy.

This Cucumber Cooler is a light and refreshing drink that is perfect for a warm day. The combination of cucumber, lime, and mint creates a delicious and hydrating drink low in sugar and perfect for those with diabetes. Enjoy this drink as a healthy alternative to sugary beverages.

Apple Cinnamon: apples, cinnamon, nutmeg

Serving size: 1 cup (240 ml)

Servings per recipe: Approximately 2

Nutritional Information per serving:

- Calories: 104
- Total Fat: 0.5 grams
- Saturated Fat: 0.1 grams
- Cholesterol: 0 milligrams
- Sodium: 2 milligrams
- Total Carbohydrates: 27 grams
- Dietary Fiber: 5 grams
- Total Sugars: 9 grams
- Protein: 0.5 grams

Ingredients:

- Four apples

- Two tablespoons of ground cinnamon

- Three tablespoons of ground nutmeg

Instructions:

1. In a Juicer or blender, combine the apple slices, cinnamon, and nutmeg.

2. Blend until mixed well.

3. Strain the juice to remove any solids.

4. Serve immediately, over ice if desired.

This Apple Cinnamon Juice is a delicious and healthy way to enjoy apples' natural sweetness without adding extra sugar. The cinnamon and nutmeg add a warm and cozy flavor, making this juice perfect for cooler months. It's a simple, tasty, and healthy option for those with diabetes. Enjoy as a tasty alternative to sugary juices.

Pineapple Punch: pineapple, Ginger, turmeric

Serving size: 1 cup (240 ml)

Servings per recipe: Approximately 2

Nutritional Information per serving:

- Calories: 130
- Total Fat: 0.7 grams
- Saturated Fat: 0.1 grams
- Cholesterol: 0 milligrams
- Sodium: 2 milligrams
- Total Carbohydrates: 33 grams
- Dietary Fiber: 3 grams
- Total Sugars: 7 grams
- Protein: 1 gram

Ingredients:

- Four cups chopped pineapple

- One piece of Ginger

- One tablespoon of turmeric powder

Instructions:

1. Combine the chopped pineapple, grated Ginger, and turmeric powder in a Juicer or blender.

2. Blend until mixed well.

3. Pour into glasses and Enjoy drinking.

This Pineapple Punch is a sweet and refreshing drink packed with flavor and nutrients. The combination of pineapple, Ginger, and turmeric makes for a delicious and healthy drink that is low in sugar and perfect for those with diabetes. Enjoy this drink as a healthy alternative to sugary beverages.

Spicy Tomato: tomatoes, jalapeno, lime, cilantro

Serving size: 1 cup (240 ml)

Servings per recipe: Approximately 2

Nutritional Information per serving:

- Calories: 43
- Total Fat: 0.4 grams
- Saturated Fat: 0.1 grams
- Cholesterol: 0 milligrams
- Sodium: 8 milligrams
- Total Carbohydrates: 10 grams
- Dietary Fiber: 3 grams
- Total Sugars: 6 grams
- Protein: 2 grams

Ingredients:

- Six tomatoes chopped
- One jalapeno pepper
- Two limes
- 1/3 cup chopped cilantro

Instructions:

1. Combine the chopped tomatoes, jalapeno, lime juice, and chopped cilantro in a Juicer or blender.

2. Blend until mixed well.

3. Strain the juice to remove any solids.

4. Serve immediately, over ice if desired.

This Spicy Tomato Juice is a refreshing and flavorful drink that is perfect for those with diabetes. Combining sweet and juicy tomatoes with spicy jalapeno, tangy lime, and fresh cilantro creates a delicious and healthy drink low in sugar. Enjoy this drink as a tasty alternative to sugary juice.

Ginger Zinger: Ginger, lemon, cayenne pepper, honey

Serving size: 1 cup (240 ml)

Servings per recipe: Approximately 1

Nutritional Information per serving:

- Calories: 44
- Total Fat: 0.1 grams
- Saturated Fat: 0 grams
- Cholesterol: 0 milligrams
- Sodium: 2 milligrams
- Total Carbohydrates: 12 grams
- Dietary Fiber: 0.2 grams
- Total Sugars: 10 grams
- Protein: 0.3 grams

Ingredients:

- Two pieces of Ginger

- Two lemons juiced

- 1/8 tablespoon cayenne pepper

- One tablespoon Sugar substitute or honey alternative (e.g. stevia, erythritol)

Instructions:

1.   In a Juicer or blender, combine the grated Ginger, lemon juice, cayenne pepper, and sugar substitute or honey alternative.

2.   Blend until mixed well.

3.   Strain the juice to remove any solids.

4.   Serve immediately over ice if desired.

This Ginger Zinger Juice is a tangy, spicy drink packed with flavor and nutrients. The combination of Ginger, lemon, cayenne pepper, and sugar substitute or honey alternative makes for a delicious and healthy drink that is low in sugar and perfect for those with diabetes. Enjoy this drink as a healthy alternative to sugary juices.

Fennel Frenzy: fennel, apples, celery, lemon

Serving size: 1 cup (240 ml)

Servings per recipe: Approximately 1

Nutritional Information per serving:

- Calories: 108
- Total Fat: 0.4 grams
- Saturated Fat: 0.1 grams
- Cholesterol: 0 milligrams
- Sodium: 73 milligrams
- Total Carbohydrates: 28 grams
- Dietary Fiber: 7 grams
- Total Sugars: 11 grams
- Protein: 2 grams

Ingredients:

- Two fennel bulbs chopped

- Two apples cored and chopped

- Two stalks of celery chopped

- One lemon juiced

Instructions:

1. Combine the chopped fennel, apples, celery, and fresh lemon juice in a Juicer or blender.

2. Blend until mixed well.

3. Strain the juice to remove any solids.

4. Serve immediately, over ice if desired.

This Fennel Frenzy Juice is a refreshing and flavorful drink packed with nutrients. The combination of fennel, apples, celery, and lemon creates a delicious and healthy drink low in sugar and perfect for those with diabetes. Enjoy this drink as a tasty alternative to sugary juices.

Green Ginger: kale, spinach, Ginger, lemon

Serving size: 1 cup (240 ml)

Servings per recipe: Approximately 1

Nutritional Information per serving:

- Calories: 46
- Total Fat: 0.4 grams
- Saturated Fat: 0.1 grams
- Cholesterol: 0 milligrams
- Sodium: 56 milligrams
- Total Carbohydrates: 11 grams
- Dietary Fiber: 3 grams
- Total Sugars: 2 grams
- Protein: 3 grams

Ingredients:

- Fresh kale leaves
- Fresh spinach leaves
- One piece of Ginger
- One lemon juiced

Instructions:

1. Combine the chopped kale, spinach, grated Ginger, and lemon juice in a Juicer or blender.

2. Blend until mixed well.

3. Strain the juice to remove any solids.

4. Serve immediately, over ice if desired.

This Green Ginger Juice is a nutrient-packed drink perfect for those with diabetes. The combination of kale, spinach, Ginger, and lemon creates a delicious and healthy drink low in sugar. Enjoy this drink as a tasty alternative to sugary juices and a great way to get your daily dose of greens.

Sweet Potato Pie: sweet potatoes, apples, cinnamon, nutmeg

Serving size: 1 cup (240 ml)

Servings per recipe: Approximately 1

Nutritional Information per serving:

- Calories: 141
- Total Fat: 0.4 grams
- Saturated Fat: 0.1 grams
- Cholesterol: 0 milligrams
- Sodium: 39 milligrams
- Total Carbohydrates: 33 grams
- Dietary Fiber: 5 grams
- Total Sugars: 4 grams
- Protein: 2 grams

Ingredients:

- Two sweet potatoes, peeled and chopped

- Two apples

- One tablespoon of cinnamon

- 1/4 tablespoon nutmeg

Instructions:

1.   Combine the chopped sweet potatoes, apples, cinnamon, and nutmeg in a Juicer or blender.

2.   Blend until mixed well.

3.   Strain the juice to remove any solids.

4.   Serve immediately, over ice if desired.

This Sweet Potato Pie Juice is a sweet and flavorful drink that is perfect for those with diabetes. The combination of sweet potatoes, apples, cinnamon, and nutmeg creates a delicious and healthy drink that is low in sugar and packed with nutrients. Enjoy this drink as a healthy alternative to sugary juices and a great way to get your daily dose of vitamins and minerals.

Rainbow Chard: rainbow chard, apples, Ginger, lemon

Serving size: 1 cup (240 ml)

Servings per recipe: Approximately 1

Nutritional Information per serving:

- Calories: 78
- Total Fat: 0.5 grams
- Saturated Fat: 0.1 grams
- Cholesterol: 0 milligrams
- Sodium: 81 milligrams
- Total Carbohydrates: 20 grams
- Dietary Fiber: 4 grams
- Total Sugars: 6 grams
- Protein: 2 grams

Ingredients:

- Two cups rainbow chard leaves chopped

- Two apples

- One piece of Ginger

- One lemon juiced

Instructions:

1.   In a Juicer or blender, combine the chopped rainbow chard, apples, grated Ginger, and lemon juice.

2.   Blend until mixed well.

3.   Strain the juice to remove any solids.

4.   Serve immediately, over ice if desired.

This Rainbow Chard Juice is a nutrient-packed drink that is perfect for those with diabetes. The combination of rainbow chard, apples, Ginger, and lemon creates a delicious and healthy drink low in sugar. Enjoy this drink as a tasty alternative to sugary juices and a great way to get your daily dose of greens.

Carrot Ginger: carrots, Ginger, lemon

Serving size: 1 cup (240 ml)

Servings per recipe: Approximately 1

Nutritional Information per serving:

- Calories: 77
- Total Fat: 0.5 grams
- Saturated Fat: 0.1 grams
- Cholesterol: 0 milligrams
- Sodium: 97 milligrams
- Total Carbohydrates: 18 grams
- Dietary Fiber: 5 grams
- Total Sugars: 9 grams
- Protein: 2 grams

Ingredients:

- Four carrots

- One piece of Ginger

- One lemon juiced

Instructions:

1. Combine the chopped carrots, grated Ginger, and lemon juice in a juicer or blender.

2. Blend until mixed well.

3. Strain the juice to remove any solids.

4. Serve immediately, over ice if desired.

This Carrot Ginger Juice is a sweet and flavorful drink that is perfect for those with diabetes. The combination of carrots, Ginger, and lemon creates a delicious and healthy drink that is low in sugar and packed with nutrients. Enjoy this drink as a healthy alternative to sugary juices and a great way to get your daily dose of vitamins and minerals.

Cucumber Melon: cucumber, cantaloupe, mint

Serving size: 1 cup (240 ml)

Servings per recipe: Approximately 1

Nutritional Information per serving:

- Calories: 83
- Total Fat: 0.5 grams
- Saturated Fat: 0.1 grams
- Cholesterol: 0 milligrams
- Sodium: 43 milligrams
- Total Carbohydrates: 20 grams
- Dietary Fiber: 3 grams
- Total Sugars: 12 grams
- Protein: 2 grams

Ingredients:

- One large cucumber

- Two cups of fresh cantaloupe

- 1/3 cup fresh mint leaves

Instructions:

1. Combine the chopped cucumber, cantaloupe, and mint leaves in a Juicer or blender.

2. Blend until mixed well.

3. Strain the juice to remove any solids.

4. Serve immediately, over ice if desired.

This Cucumber Melon Juice is a sweet and refreshing drink that is perfect for those with diabetes. The combination of cucumber, cantaloupe, and mint creates a delicious and healthy drink low in sugar and packed with nutrients. Enjoy this drink as a healthy alternative to sugary juices and a great way to get your daily dose of vitamins and minerals.

Sweet Pea: frozen peas, mint, lemon

Serving size: 1 cup (240 ml)

Servings per recipe: Approximately 1

Nutritional Information per serving:

- Calories: 82
- Total Fat: 0.6 grams
- Saturated Fat: 0.1 grams
- Cholesterol: 0 milligrams
- Sodium: 167 milligrams
- Total Carbohydrates: 15 grams
- Dietary Fiber: 5 grams
- Total Sugars: 5 grams
- Protein: 5 grams

Ingredients:

- Two cups frozen peas
- 1/3 cup mint leaves
- One lemon juiced

Instructions:

1. Combine the frozen green peas, mint leaves, and lemon juice in a Juicer or blender.
2. Blend until mixed well.
3. Strain the juice to remove any solids.
4. Serve immediately, over ice if desired.

This Sweet Pea Juice is a fresh and flavorful drink that is perfect for those with diabetes. The combination of green peas, mint, and lemon creates a delicious and healthy drink low in sugar and packed with nutrients. Enjoy this drink as a healthy alternative to sugary juices and a great way to get your daily dose of vitamins and minerals.

Orange Carrot: carrots, oranges, Ginger, turmeric

Serving size: 1 cup (240 ml)

Servings per recipe: Approximately 1

Nutritional Information per serving:

- Calories: 105
- Total Fat: 0.5 grams
- Saturated Fat: 0.1 grams
- Cholesterol: 0 milligrams
- Sodium: 56 milligrams
- Total Carbohydrates: 26 grams
- Dietary Fiber: 6 grams
- Total Sugars: 8 grams
- Protein: 2 grams

Ingredients:

- Four carrots
- Two oranges
- One piece of Ginger
- 1/2 teaspoon turmeric powder

Instructions:

1. In a Juicer or blender, combine the chopped carrots, oranges, grated Ginger, and turmeric powder.

2. Blend until mixed well.

3. Strain the juice to remove any solids.

4. Serve immediately, over ice if desired.

This Orange Carrot Juice is a sweet and flavorful drink that is perfect for those with diabetes. Combining carrots, oranges, Ginger, and turmeric creates a delicious and healthy drink that is low in sugar and packed with nutrients. Enjoy this drink as a healthy alternative to sugary juices and a great way to get your daily dose of vitamins and minerals.

Pineapple Mint: pineapple, mint, lime

Serving size: 1 cup (240 ml)

Servings per recipe: Approximately 1

Nutritional Information per serving:

- Calories: 94
- Total Fat: 0.6 grams
- Saturated Fat: 0.1 grams
- Cholesterol: 0 milligrams
- Sodium: 2 milligrams
- Total Carbohydrates: 24 grams
- Dietary Fiber: 2 grams
- Total Sugars: 7 grams
- Protein: 1 gram

Ingredients:

- Two cups pineapple chopped

- 1/3 cup mint leaves

- One lime juiced

Instructions:

1. Combine the chopped pineapple, mint leaves, and lime juice in a Juicer or blender.

2. Blend until mixed well.

3. Strain the juice to remove any solids.

4. Serve immediately, over ice if desired.

This Pineapple Mint Juice is a sweet and refreshing drink that is perfect for those with diabetes. The combination of pineapple, mint, and lime creates a delicious and healthy drink low in sugar and packed with nutrients. Enjoy this drink as a healthy alternative to sugary juices and a great way to get your daily dose of vitamins and minerals.

Green Glory: kale, spinach, cucumber, celery, parsley, lemon

Serving size: 1 cup (240 ml)

Servings per recipe: Approximately 1

Nutritional Information per serving:

- Calories: 40
- Total Fat: 0.5 grams
- Saturated Fat: 0.1 grams
- Cholesterol: 0 milligrams
- Sodium: 58 milligrams
- Total Carbohydrates: 9 grams
- Dietary Fiber: 3 grams
- Total Sugars: 3 grams
- Protein: 3 grams

Ingredients:

- Two cups fresh kale chopped
- Two cups green spinach chopped
- One large cucumber peeled and chopped
- Two stalks of celery chopped
- 1/4 cup parsley leaves
- One lemon juiced

Instructions:

1. Combine the chopped kale, spinach, cucumber, celery, parsley, and lemon juice in a Juicer or blender.

2. Blend until mixed well.

3. Strain the juice to remove any solids.

4. Serve immediately, over ice if desired.

This Green Glory Juice is a nutritious and delicious drink that is perfect for those with diabetes. Combining kale, spinach, cucumber, celery, parsley, and lemon creates a healthy drink low in sugar and packed with vitamins and minerals. Enjoy this drink as a healthy alternative to sugary juices and a great way to get your daily dose of greens.

Carrot Apple: carrots, apples, Ginger

Serving size: 1 cup (240 ml)

Servings per recipe: Approximately 1

Nutritional Information per serving:

- Calories: 75
- Total Fat: 0.3 grams
- Saturated Fat: 0 grams
- Cholesterol: 0 milligrams
- Sodium: 50 milligrams
- Total Carbohydrates: 18 grams
- Dietary Fiber: 4 grams
- Total Sugars: 12 grams
- Protein: 1 gram

Ingredients:

- Four carrots, peeled and chopped

- Two apples, cored and chopped

- One piece of Ginger

Instructions:

1. In a Juicer or blender, combine the chopped carrots, apples, and grated Ginger.

2. Blend until mixed well.

3. Strain the juice to remove any solids.

4. Serve immediately, over ice if desired.

This Carrot Apple Juice is a sweet and flavorful drink that is perfect for those with diabetes. The combination of carrots, apples and Ginger creates a delicious and healthy drink low in sugar and packed with nutrients. Enjoy this drink as a healthy alternative to sugary juices and a great way to get your daily dose of vitamins and minerals. Ginger adds a spicy and aromatic flavor that complements the sweetness of the carrots and apples.

Beet Blast: beets, carrots, apples, Ginger

Serving size: 1 cup (240 ml)

Servings per recipe: Approximately 1

Nutritional Information per serving:

- Calories: 105
- Total Fat: 0.5 grams
- Saturated Fat: 0.1 grams
- Cholesterol: 0 milligrams
- Sodium: 85 milligrams
- Total Carbohydrates: 25 grams
- Dietary Fiber: 6 grams
- Total Sugars: 10 grams
- Protein: 2 grams

Ingredients:

- Two beets, peeled and chopped
- Fourcarrots, peeled and chopped
- Two apples
- One piece of Ginger

Instructions:

1. Combine the chopped beets, carrots, apples, and grated Ginger in a Juicer or blender.
2. Blend until mixed well.
3. Strain the juice to remove any solids.
4. Serve immediately, over ice if desired.

This Beet Blast Juice is a sweet and earthy drink that is perfect for those with diabetes. The combination of beets, carrots, apples, and Ginger creates a delicious and healthy drink low in sugar and packed with nutrients. Enjoy this drink as a healthy alternative to sugary juices and a great way to get your daily dose of vitamins and minerals. The beets add a sweet and earthy flavor to the drink, while the carrots, apples, and Ginger provide additional sweetness and flavor.

Citrus Kick: grapefruit, oranges, lemons, limes, mint

Serving size: 1 cup (240 ml)

Servings per recipe: Approximately 1

Nutritional Information per serving:

- Calories: 110
- Total Fat: 0.3 grams
- Saturated Fat: 0 grams
- Cholesterol: 0 milligrams
- Sodium: 2 milligrams
- Total Carbohydrates: 28 grams
- Dietary Fiber: 6 grams
- Total Sugars: 8 grams
- Protein: 2 grams

Ingredients:

- One large grapefruit, peeled and chopped
- Two oranges, peeled and chopped
- One lemon juiced
- One lime juiced
- 1/3 cup mint leaves

Instructions:

1. Combine the chopped grapefruit, oranges, lemon juice, lime juice, and mint leaves in a Juicer or blender.

2. Blend until mixed well.

3. Strain the juice to remove any solids.

4. Serve immediately, over ice if desired.

This Citrus Kick Juice is a refreshing and tangy drink that is perfect for those with diabetes. The combination of grapefruit, oranges, lemon, lime, and mint creates a delicious and healthy drink low in sugar and packed with vitamins and minerals. Enjoy this drink as a healthy alternative to sugary juices and a great way to get your daily dose of citrus. The mint adds a fresh and cooling flavor that complements the tangy and sweet flavors of citrus fruits.

Cucumber Lime: cucumber, lime, mint

Serving size: 1 cup (240 ml)

Servings per recipe: Approximately 1

Nutritional Information per serving:

- Calories: 11
- Total Fat: 0.1 grams
- Saturated Fat: 0 grams
- Cholesterol: 0 milligrams
- Sodium: 2 milligrams
- Total Carbohydrates: 3 grams
- Dietary Fiber: 1 gram
- Total Sugars: 1 gram
- Protein: 0.5 grams

Ingredients:

- Two cucumbers, peeled and chopped
- Two limes juiced
- 1/3 cup mint leaves

Instructions:

1. Combine the chopped cucumbers, lime juice, and mint leaves in a Juicer or blender.

2. Blend until mixed well.

3. Strain the juice to remove any solids.

4. Serve immediately, over ice if desired.

This Cucumber Lime Juice is a refreshing and hydrating drink that is perfect for those with diabetes. The combination of cucumbers, lime, and mint creates a delicious and healthy drink low in sugar and packed with vitamins and minerals. Enjoy this drink as a healthy alternative to sugary juices and a great way to stay hydrated. The cucumbers provide a fresh and crisp flavor, while the lime adds a tangy and sweet taste. The mint adds a fresh and cooling flavor that perfectly complements the cucumbers and lime.

Apple Pie: apples, cinnamon, nutmeg

Serving size: 1 cup (240 ml)

Servings per recipe: Approximately 1

Nutritional Information per serving:

- Calories: 120
- Total Fat: 0.5 grams
- Saturated Fat: 0.1 grams
- Cholesterol: 0 milligrams
- Sodium: 1 milligram
- Total Carbohydrates: 31 grams
- Dietary Fiber: 5 grams
- Total Sugars: 4 grams
- Protein: 1 gram

Ingredients:

- Four apples

- one tablespoon of freshly ground cinnamon

- Two tablespoons of ground nutmeg

Instructions:

1. In a Juicer or blender, combine the chopped apples, cinnamon, and nutmeg.

2. Blend until mixed well.

3. Strain the juice to remove any solids.

4. Serve immediately, over ice if desired.

This Apple Pie Juice is a delicious and healthy drink that tastes just like your favorite dessert! The combination of apples, cinnamon, and nutmeg creates a sweet and spicy flavor that is perfect for those with diabetes. The apples provide a sweet and juicy flavor, while the cinnamon and nutmeg add a warm and spicy taste. This drink is the perfect way to enjoy the flavors of apple pie without the added sugar.

Pineapple Paradise: pineapple, coconut water, mint

Serving size: 1 cup (240 ml)

Servings per recipe: Approximately 1

Nutritional Information per serving:

- Calories: 130
- Total Fat: 0.5 grams
- Saturated Fat: 0 grams
- Cholesterol: 0 milligrams
- Sodium: 100 milligrams
- Total Carbohydrates: 33 grams
- Dietary Fiber: 4 grams
- Total Sugars: 2 grams
- Protein: 2 grams

Ingredients:

- Four cups pineapple chopped
- Two cups of coconut water
- 1/3 cup mint leaves

Instructions:

1. Combine the chopped pineapple, coconut water, and mint leaves in a Juicer or blender.
2. Blend until mixed well.
3. Strain the juice to remove any solids.
4. Serve immediately, over ice if desired.

This Pineapple Paradise Juice is a delicious and healthy drink that is perfect for those with diabetes. The combination of pineapple, coconut water, and mint creates a refreshing and tropical flavor low in sugar and packed with vitamins and minerals. Enjoy this drink as a healthy alternative to sugary juices and a great way to stay hydrated. The pineapple provides a sweet and juicy flavor, while the coconut water adds a refreshing and hydrating taste. The mint adds a fresh and cooling flavor that perfectly complements the pineapple and coconut water.

Tomato Tango: tomatoes, red bell peppers, jalapenos, lime

Serving size: 1 cup (240 ml)

Servings per recipe: Approximately 1

Nutritional Information per serving:

- Calories: 50
- Total Fat: 0.5 grams
- Saturated Fat: 0 grams
- Cholesterol: 0 milligrams
- Sodium: 10 milligrams
- Total Carbohydrates: 12 grams
- Dietary Fiber: 4 grams
- Total Sugars: 7 grams
- Protein: 2 grams

Ingredients:

- Four tomatoes chopped

- One red bell pepper

- One small jalapeno pepper

- One lime juiced

Instructions:

Combine the chopped tomatoes, red bell pepper, jalapeno, and lime juice in a Juicer or blender.

1. Blend until mixed well.

2. Strain the juice to remove any solids.

3. Serve immediately, over ice if desired.

This Tomato Tango Juice is a delicious and healthy drink that is perfect for those with diabetes. The combination of tomatoes, red bell pepper, jalapeno, and lime creates a spicy and tangy flavor low in sugar and packed with vitamins and minerals. The tomatoes provide a sweet and juicy flavor, while the red bell pepper adds a mild and sweet taste. The jalapeno and lime add a spicy and tangy flavor that perfectly complements the tomatoes and red bell pepper's sweetness.

Ginger Gold: Ginger, lemon, honey, turmeric

Serving size: 1 cup (240 ml)

Servings per recipe: Approximately 1

Nutritional Information per serving:

- Calories: 80
- Total Fat: 0 g
- Saturated Fat: 0 g
- Trans Fat: 0 g
- Cholesterol: 0 mg
- Sodium: 3 mg
- Total Carbohydrates: 21 g
- Dietary Fiber: 1 g
- Sugars: 7 g
- Protein: 0 g

Ingredients:

- One-inch fresh ginger root, peeled and chopped
- One lemon juiced
- One tablespoon of honey
- 1/2 teaspoon turmeric

Instructions:

1. Combine the chopped Ginger, lemon juice, honey, and turmeric in a Juicer or blender.
2. Blend until mixed well.
3. Strain the juice to remove any solids.
4. Serve immediately, over ice if desired.

This Ginger Gold Juice is a delicious and healthy drink that is perfect for those with diabetes. The combination of Ginger, lemon, honey, and turmeric creates a spicy and sweet flavor that is low in sugar and packed with vitamins and minerals. Enjoy this drink as a healthy alternative to sugary juices and a great way to boost your immune system. The Ginger provides a spicy and zesty flavor, while the lemon adds a tangy and sour taste. The honey and turmeric add a sweet and warming flavor that perfectly complements the Ginger's spiciness and the sourness of the lemon. Please note while honey is a natural sweetener, it should still be consumed in moderation by those with diabetes.

Fennel Fresh: fennel, apples, celery, mint

Serving size: 1 cup (240 ml)

Servings per recipe: Approximately 1

Nutritional Information per serving:

- Calories: 45
- Total Fat: 0 g
- Saturated Fat: 0 g
- Trans Fat: 0 g
- Cholesterol: 0 mg
- Sodium: 75 mg
- Total Carbohydrates: 11 g
- Dietary Fiber: 3 g
- Sugars: 6 g
- Protein: 1 g

Ingredients:

- One -sized fennel bulb, chopped

- Two apples, cored and chopped

- Two stalks of celery, chopped

- 1/4 cup fresh mint leaves

Instructions:

1. Combine the chopped fennel, apples, celery, and mint leaves in a Juicer or blender.

2. Blend until mixed well.

3. Strain the juice to remove any solids.

4. Serve immediately, over ice if desired.

This Fennel Fresh Juice is a delicious and healthy drink that is perfect for those with diabetes. The combination of fennel, apples, celery, and mint creates a refreshing and crisp flavor low in sugar and packed with vitamins and minerals. Enjoy this drink as a healthy alternative to sugary juices and a great way to boost your immune system. The fennel provides a licorice-like flavor, while the apples and celery add a sweet and crisp taste. The mint leaves add a fresh and cooling flavor that perfectly complements the apples and celery's sweetness.

Green Grape: kale, spinach, grapes, lemon

Serving size: 1 cup (240 ml)

Servings per recipe: Approximately 1

Nutritional Information per serving:

- Calories: 70
- Total Fat: 0.5 g
- Saturated Fat: 0 g
- Trans Fat: 0 g
- Cholesterol: 0 mg
- Sodium: 39 mg
- Total Carbohydrates: 17 g
- Dietary Fiber: 3 g
- Sugars: 10 g
- Protein: 3 g

Ingredients:

- Two cups freshly chopped kale

- Two cups freshly chopped spinach

- Three cups red grapes seeded

- One lemon peeled

Instructions:

1. Combine the chopped kale, spinach, grapes, and lemon in a Juicer or blender.

2. Blend until mixed well.

3. Strain the juice to remove any solids.

4. Serve immediately, over ice if desired.

This Green Grape Juice is a sweet and healthy drink that is perfect for those with diabetes. The combination of kale, spinach, grapes, and lemon creates a sweet and tangy flavor low in sugar and packed with vitamins and minerals. The kale and spinach are great sources of fiber and antioxidants, while the grapes provide a natural sweetness that helps to satisfy sugar cravings. The lemon provides a zesty flavor that helps to balance out the sweetness of the grapes and adds a burst of vitamin C. Enjoy this drink as a healthy alternative to sugary juices and a great way to boost your immune system.

Sweet Spice: sweet potatoes, apples, cinnamon, nutmeg, allspice

Serving size: 1 cup (240 ml)

Servings per recipe: Approximately 1

Nutritional Information per serving:

- Calories: 155
- Total Fat: 0.5 g
- Saturated Fat: 0 g
- Trans Fat: 0 g
- Cholesterol: 0 mg
- Sodium: 51 mg
- Total Carbohydrates: 38 g
- Dietary Fiber: 5 g
- Sugars: 8 g
- Protein: 2 g

Ingredients:

- Two sweet potatoes, peeled and chopped

- Two apples

- One tablespoon cinnamon

- Two tablespoon nutmeg

- 1/4 tablespoon allspice

Instructions:

1.   Combine the chopped sweet potatoes, apples, cinnamon, nutmeg, and allspice in a Juicer or blender.

2.   Blend until mixed well.

3.   Strain the juice to remove any solids.

4.   Serve immediately, over ice if desired.

This Sweet Spice Juice is a warming and delicious drink that is perfect for those with diabetes. The combination of sweet potatoes, apples, cinnamon, nutmeg, and allspice creates a sweet and spicy flavor low in sugar and packed with nutrients. Enjoy this drink as a healthy alternative to sugary juices and a great way to boost your energy levels.

Rainbow Twist: rainbow chard, apples, Ginger, lemon, mint

Serving size: 1 cup (240 ml)

Servings per recipe: Approximately 1

Nutritional Information per serving:

- Calories: 70
- Total Fat: 0.5 g
- Saturated Fat: 0 g
- Trans Fat: 0 g
- Cholesterol: 0 mg
- Sodium: 48 mg
- Total Carbohydrates: 18 g
- Dietary Fiber: 3 g
- Sugars: 10 g
- Protein: 2 g

Ingredients:

- Two cups rainbow chard washed and chopped

- Two apples

- A one-inch piece of Ginger, peeled and chopped

- One lemon

- 1/4 cup fresh mint leaves

Instructions:

1.   In a Juicer or blender, combine the chopped rainbow chard, apples, Ginger, lemon, and mint.

2.   Blend until mixed well.

3.   Strain the juice to remove any solids.

4.   Serve immediately, over ice if desired.

This Rainbow Twist Juice is a healthy and flavorful drink that is perfect for people with diabetes. Enjoy this drink as a healthy alternative to sugary juices and a great way to boost your energy levels.

Carrot Kick: carrots, Ginger, lemon, cayenne pepper

Serving size: 1 cup (240 ml)

Servings per recipe: Approximately 1

Nutritional Information per serving:

- Calories: 70
- Total Fat: 0.5 g
- Saturated Fat: 0 g
- Trans Fat: 0 g
- Cholesterol: 0 mg
- Sodium: 82 mg
- Total Carbohydrates: 16 g
- Dietary Fiber: 4 g
- Sugars: 8 g
- Protein: 2 g

Ingredients:

- Two cups carrots, peeled and chopped
- A one-inch piece of Ginger, peeled and chopped
- One lemon, peeled and seeded
- 1/4 teaspoon cayenne pepper

Instructions:

1. Combine the chopped carrots, Ginger, lemon, and cayenne pepper in a Juicer or blender.

2. Blend until mixed well.

3. Strain the juice to remove any solids.

4. Serve immediately, over ice if desired.

This Carrot Kick Juice is a healthy and flavorful drink that is perfect for people with diabetes. Carrots are a unique source of vitamins, minerals, and fiber, while Ginger and lemon add a zesty flavor that helps balance the carrots' sweetness. The cayenne pepper provides a kick of heat that helps to boost metabolism and increase energy levels. Enjoy this drink as a healthy alternative to sugary juices and a great way to start your day.

Cucumber Cuke: cucumber, lime, honeydew melon

Serving size: 1 cup (240 ml)

Servings per recipe: Approximately 1

Nutritional Information per serving:

- Calories: 110
- Total Fat: 0.5 g
- Saturated Fat: 0 g
- Trans Fat: 0 g
- Cholesterol: 0 mg
- Sodium: 55 mg
- Total Carbohydrates: 27 g
- Dietary Fiber: 3
- Sugars: 1 g
- Protein: 1 g

Ingredients:

- Two cups cucumber, peeled and chopped

- One lime, peeled and seeded

- Two cups honeydew melon, peeled and chopped

Instructions:

1. Combine the chopped cucumber, lime, and honeydew melon in a Juicer or blender.

2. Blend until mixed well.

3. Strain the juice to remove any solids.

4. Serve immediately, over ice if desired.

This Cucumber Cuke Juice is a refreshing and hydrating drink that is perfect for people with diabetes. Cucumber is an excellent source of hydration and helps to cleanse the body, while lime adds a zesty flavor that helps to balance out the sweetness of the honeydew melon. Honeydew melon is an excellent source of vitamin C and potassium. Enjoy this drink as a healthy alternative to sugary juices and a great way to stay hydrated throughout the day.

Sweet Sip: frozen peas, mint, lemon, honey

Serving size: 1 cup (240 ml)

Servings per recipe: Approximately 1

Nutritional Information per serving:

- Calories: 110
- Total Fat: 0.5 g
- Saturated Fat: 0 g
- Trans Fat: 0 g
- Cholesterol: 0 mg
- Sodium: 45 mg
- Total Carbohydrates: 27 g
- Dietary Fiber: 4 g
- Sugars: 9 g
- Protein: 3 g

Ingredients:

- Two cups frozen peas

- One lemon

- 1/3 cup fresh mint leaves

- One tablespoon honey (optional)

Instructions:

1. In a Juicer or blender, combine the frozen peas, lemon, mint leaves, and honey (if using).

2. Blend until mixed well.

3. Strain the juice to remove any solids.

4. Serve immediately, over ice if desired.

This Sweet Sip Juice is a delicious and healthy drink that is perfect for people with diabetes. Frozen peas are an excellent source of protein and fiber, while lemon provides a zesty flavor that helps maintain the drink's sweetness. Mint adds a refreshing flavor and provides a boost of antioxidants that help to improve overall health. The optional honey can be used to add a touch of sweetness, but it is not necessary for a delicious and healthy drink. Enjoy this Sweet Sip Juice as a healthy alternative to sugary juices and a great way to stay hydrated throughout the day.

Orange Oasis: carrots, oranges, Ginger, honey

Ingredients:

- Two carrots

- Two oranges

- One piece of Ginger

- One tablespoon honey (optional)

Instructions:

1. In a Juicer or blender, combine the carrots, oranges, Ginger, and honey (if using).

2. Blend until mixed well.

3. Strain the juice to remove any solids.

4. Serve immediately, over ice if desired.

This Orange Oasis Juice is a delicious and healthy drink that is perfect for people with diabetes. Enjoy this Orange Oasis Juice as a healthy alternative to sugary juices and a great way to stay hydrated throughout the day.

Apple Juice Detox

Serving size: 1 cup (240 ml)

Servings per recipe: Approximately 1

Nutritional Information per serving:

- Calories: 60
- Total Fat: 0.5 g
- Saturated Fat: 0 g
- Trans Fat: 0 g
- Cholesterol: 0 mg
- Sodium: 40 mg
- Total Carbohydrates: 15 g
- Dietary Fiber: 2 g
- Sugars: 10 g
- Protein: 1 g

Ingredients

- ½ cup green apples

- ½ cup mint leaves

- one lemon

- one orange

- one cucumber

Instructions

1.	In a juicer, begin by juicing the apples and mint, then the lemon and orange, and finally, the cucumber.

2.	Combine everything by giving it a thorough stir.

3.	If you are using a juicer or blender, add all of the ingredients and purée them until they are smooth.

4.	Enjoy drinking!

Dandy-Kale Delight

Serving size: 1 cup (240 ml)

Servings per recipe: Approximately 1

Nutritional Information per serving:

- Calories: 146
- Total fat: 1g
- Saturated fat: 0g
- Trans fat: 0g
- Cholesterol: 0mg
- Sodium: 95mg
- Total carbohydrates: 35g
- Dietary fiber: 5g
- Sugars: 9 g
- Protein: 4g

Ingredients

- ½ cup dandelion greens
- ½ cup kale leaves
- ¼ cup parsley
- 1 cup cucumber
- ½ cup celery

Instructions

1.   Using a juicer, begin by processing the dandelion greens, kale, and parsley, followed by the cucumber and celery. Combine everything by giving it a thorough stir. Put all ingredients in a juicer or blender, and process them until they form a homogeneous paste.

2.   Enjoy sipping!

The vibrant green color of this beverage gives you an idea of the health advantages provided by the substances it contains.

Italian Fennel Cleanse

Servings per recipe: Approximately 1

Nutritional Information per serving:

- Calories: 84
- Total fat: 0.5g
- Saturated fat: 0g
- Trans fat: 0g
- Cholesterol: 0mg
- Sodium: 48mg
- Total carbohydrates: 21g
- Dietary fiber: 3g
- Sugars: 15g
- Protein: 2g

Ingredients

- ¼ cup garlic cloves, peeled

- ½ cup fennel

- ½ cup kale leaves

- Eight basil leaves

- ½ cup tomatoes

- ¼ cup cucumber

- One lemon

Instructions

1.   In a juicer, first process the garlic cloves, fennel, kale, and basil. Next, add the tomatoes, cucumber, and lemon.

2.   Process until smooth.

3.   Combine everything by giving it a thorough stir. If you use a juicer or blender, add all ingredients and purée until completely smooth.

This beverage has a peppery flavor thanks to the fennel, balanced out by the citrusy freshness of the lemon juice. Together, these ingredients work to detoxify your body.

The Delicious Green Cleanse

Serving size: 1 cup (240 ml)

Servings per recipe: Approximately 1

Nutritional Information per serving:

- Calories: 140
- Total fat: 1g
- Saturated fat: 0g
- Trans fat: 0g
- Cholesterol: 0mg
- Sodium: 104mg
- Total carbohydrates: 34g
- Dietary fiber: 5g
- Sugars: 12g
- Protein: 3g

Ingredients

- ½ cup green bell peppers

- ¼ cup broccoli florets

- ½ cup cucumber

- ½ cup cabbage

Instructions

1.	Start by juicing the bell peppers and broccoli in a juicer, then move on to the cucumber and cabbage.

2.	Combine everything by giving it a thorough stir. Put all ingredients in a juicer or blender, and process them until they form a homogeneous paste.

3.	Enjoy drinking.

This vibrant green beverage is just as healthy for you as it appears. The good news is that it has a pleasant and reviving flavor despite its powerful ability to protect against sickness and purify the body. Each component functions admirably when used by itself, but when combined, they form a formidable force. If you find this beverage's flavor is too heavy, try adding a little extra cucumber.

Ingredients

- One cup spinach

- One lemon

- ¼ cup parsley

- ½ cup celery

Instructions

1.   The spinach and the lemon should be juiced first, followed by the parsley and the celery. Combine everything by giving it a thorough stir.

2.   If you use a juicer or blender, add all ingredients and purée until completely smooth.

3.   Enjoy sipping!

Your body will benefit from the cleansing Power of this nutrient-dense green beverage. The lemon and celery contribute a refreshing flavor while also helping to cleanse the palate, which helps keep the spinach in check.

Cabbage Soup Juice

Serving size: 1 cup (240 ml)

Servings per recipe: Approximately 1

Nutritional Information per serving:

- Calories: 50
- Total fat: 0.5 g
- Saturated fat: 0 g
- Trans fat: 0 g
- Cholesterol: 0 mg
- Sodium: 260 mg
- Total Carbohydrates: 12 g
- Dietary fiber: 4 g
- Sugars: 7 g

Ingredients

- ½ cup green cabbage
- ¼ cup garlic cloves, peeled
- 6 to 8 basil leaves
- ½ cup tomatoes
- ½ cup green bell peppers

Instructions

1. First, use a juicer to blend the cabbage, garlic cloves, and fresh basil, and then move on to the tomatoes and bell peppers.

2. Combine everything by giving it a thorough stir. Put all ingredients in a juicer or blender, and process them until they form a homogeneous paste.

3. Enjoy drinking.

Skinny Salsa Sauce

Serving size: 1 cup (240 ml)

Servings per recipe: Approximately 1

Nutritional Information per serving:

- Calories: 10
- Total fat: 0 g
- Saturated fat: 0 g
- Trans fat: 0 g
- Cholesterol: 0 mg
- Sodium: 50 mg
- Total Carbohydrates: 3 g
- Dietary fiber: 1 g
- Sugars: 2 g
- Protein: 0 g

Ingredients

- ¼ cup green onions

- ¼ cup wheatgrass

- ¼ cup lemongrass

- ¼ cup cilantro

- One cup tomatoes

- One lime

Instructions

1.   In a juicer, begin by juicing the green onions, wheatgrass, and lemongrass. Next, add the cilantro, and finish with the tomatoes and lime.

2.   Combine everything by giving it a thorough stir.

3.   If you use a blender, add all and purée until completely smooth.

This delicious juice has a low-calorie count, is fantastic for cleansing and detoxifying your entire system, and contains many of the same veggies used to make salsa. As a result, your metabolism will work more effectively. The increased oxygen consumption resulting from a high chlorophyll intake makes it easier for your body to shed unhealthily stored fat quickly. Note: If your juicer cannot process grasses, do not include them in your juice.

Vegetable Soup Juice

Serving size: 1 cup (240 ml)

Servings per recipe: Approximately 1

Nutritional Information per serving:

- Calories: 70
- Total fat: 0.5 g
- Saturated fat: 0 g
- Trans fat: 0 g
- Cholesterol: 0 mg
- Sodium: 650 mg
- Total Carbohydrates: 16 g
- Dietary fiber: 4 g
- Sugars: 7 g
- Protein: 2 g

Ingredients

- ¼ cup potatoes
- ¼ cup green onions
- 1 cup tomatoes
- ½ cup green bell peppers
- ¼ teaspoon black pepper
- Pinch of cayenne pepper

Instructions

1. First, the tomatoes and the bell peppers go through the juicer, followed by the potatoes and the onions.

2. After adding the black and cayenne peppers, give the juice a good toss to integrate everything.

3. Put all ingredients in a juicer or blender, and process them until they form a homogeneous paste.

Even if you have diabetes, you may still enjoy a mini-fast with this delicious drink, which is perfect for getting your dieting efforts off to a good start. The cayenne pepper provides an extra kick stimulating the metabolism even further.

Perfect Pepper Picker-Upper

Serving size: 1 cup (240 ml)

Servings per recipe: Approximately 1

Nutritional Information per serving:

- Calories: 90
- Total fat: 1 g
- Saturated fat: 0 g
- Trans fat: 0 g
- Cholesterol: 0 mg
- Sodium: 350 mg
- Total Carbohydrates: 22 g
- Dietary fiber: 3 g
- Sugars: 6 g
- Protein: 2 g

Ingredients

- ½ jalapeño pepper
- ½ cup green bell peppers
- ½ cup cucumber
- ½ cup arugula

Instructions

1. First, put the jalapeno and the bell peppers into the juicer, followed by the cucumber and the arugula.

2. Combine everything by giving it a thorough stir.

3. Using a juicer or blender, add all the ingredients and puree until smooth.

Serving size: 1 cup (240 ml)

Servings per recipe: Approximately 1

Nutritional Information per serving:

- Calories: 120
- Total fat: 1 g
- Saturated fat: 0 g
- Trans fat: 0 g
- Cholesterol: 0 mg
- Sodium: 480 mg
- Total Carbohydrates: 24 g
- Dietary fiber: 4 g
- Sugars: 10 g
- Protein: 6 g

Ingredients

- ¼ cup garlic cloves, peeled

- ¼ cup green bell peppers

- Six basil leaves

- One cup tomatoes

Instructions

1.   First, the garlic cloves and the peppers should be juiced in a juicer, followed by the basil and the tomatoes.

2.   Combine everything by giving it a thorough stir.

3.   Put all ingredients in a small blender, and process them until they form a homogeneous paste.

Antioxidant Ale

Serving size: 1 cup (240 ml)

Servings per recipe: Approximately 1

Nutritional Information per serving:

- Calories: 110
- Total fat: 0 g
- Saturated fat: 0 g
- Trans fat: 0 g
- Cholesterol: 0 mg
- Sodium: 25 mg
- Total Carbohydrates: 27 g
- Dietary fiber: 3 g
- Sugars: 8 g
- Protein: 2 g

Ingredients

- ¼ cup raspberries

- ¼ cup oranges

- ¼ cup strawberries

- Four mint sprigs, optional

- ¼ cup cucumber

Instructions

1. Run all of the ingredients through a juicer or blender, then swirl the juice well to combine everything.

2. If you use a blender, add all ingredients, and purée until completely smooth.

This is an excellent juice to start your day with since it tastes incredible, and the antioxidant power it packs is completely unmatched! The fruit also provides a pleasant boost to one's energy levels.

Super Shake

Serving size: 1 cup (240 ml)

Servings per recipe: Approximately 1

Nutritional Information per serving:

- Calories: 400
- Total fat: 16 g
- Saturated fat: 2 g
- Trans fat: 0 g
- Cholesterol: 0 mg
- Sodium: 230 mg
- Total Carbohydrates: 53 g
- Dietary fiber: 10 g
- Sugars: 3 g
- Protein: 20 g

Ingredients

- One head of garlic cloves, peeled
- ½ cup cabbage
- ½ cup kale leaves
- ½ cup beets
- ½ cup carrots
- ½ cup celery

Instructions

1.   Utilizing the juicer, process the garlic cloves, cabbage, and kale, move on to the carrots and beets, and then finish with the celery.

2.   Combine everything by giving it a thorough stir.

3.   Put all ingredients in a juicer or blender, and process them until they form a homogeneous paste.

Garlic cloves, kale, beets, and carrots are "super" nutrients that can help your body fight off sickness and maintain a healthy level of nutrition. You can add a pinch or two if you want to give the juice an extra antioxidant boost from the capsaicin in cayenne pepper.

Serving size: 1 cup (240 ml)

Servings per recipe: Approximately 1

Nutritional Information per serving:

- Calories: 260
- Total fat: 6 g
- Saturated fat: 1 g
- Trans fat: 0 g
- Cholesterol: 0 mg
- Sodium: 85 mg
- Total Carbohydrates: 45 g
- Dietary fiber: 7 g
- Sugars: 6 g
- Protein: 5g

Ingredients

- ½ cup green apples
- ½ cup pumpkin
- ½ cup cucumber
- ½ cup carrots
- ½ teaspoon ground cloves
- ½ teaspoon ground cinnamon

Instructions

1. Using the juicer, process the apples and pumpkin, then move on to the cucumber and carrots.

2. Add garlic cloves and cinnamon to the juice, and then give it a good toss to mix the flavors.

3. Put all ingredients in a juicer or blender, and process them until they form a homogeneous paste.

Because of how tasty it is, you won't believe this is healthy for you, but you can take my word for it because it is!

Arugula Pepper Punch

Serving size: 1 cup (240 ml)

Servings per recipe: Approximately 1

Nutritional Information per serving:

- Calories: 130
- Total fat: 1 g
- Saturated fat: 0 g
- Trans fat: 0 g
- Cholesterol: 0 mg
- Sodium: 180 mg
- Total Carbohydrates: 30 g
- Dietary fiber: 6 g
- Sugars: 6 g
- Protein: 4 g

Ingredients

- 1 cup arugula

- ¼ cup watercress

- ½ cup celery

- ½ cup lemongrass

- ¼ cup green bell peppers

- ½ teaspoon prepared horseradish

Instructions

1.   A juicer should process the arugula, watercress, and celery first, then add lemongrass and red bell peppers.

2.   After adding the horseradish to your delicious juice, please give it a nice toss to incorporate everything.

3.   Put all ingredients in a juicer or blender, and process them until they form a homogeneous paste.

Rabbit Juice

Serving size: 1 cup (240 ml)

Servings per recipe: Approximately 1

Nutritional Information per serving:

- Calories: 62
- Total fat: 0.4 g
- Saturated fat: 0.1 g
- Trans fat: 0 g
- Cholesterol: 0 mg
- Sodium: 60 mg
- Total carbohydrates: 15 g
- Dietary fiber: 3.6 g
- Sugars: 9 g
- Protein: 2.5 g

Ingredients

- One cup carrots

- ½ cup green apples

- ½ cup cucumber

- ½ cup kale leaves

Instructions

1. Process all the ingredients mentioned above in a Juicer or blender, and stir well to combine.

Potato Head juice

Serving size: 1 cup (240 ml)

Servings per recipe: Approximately 1

Nutritional Information per serving:

- Calories: 28
- Total fat: 0.2 g
- Saturated fat: 0 g
- Trans fat: 0 g
- Cholesterol: 0 mg
- Sodium: 18 mg
- Total carbohydrates: 6.5 g
- Dietary fiber: 1.8 g
- Sugars: 3.5 g
- Protein: 1.4 g

Ingredients

- One cup potatoes

- Six basil leaves

- One cup tomatoes

Instructions

1.   Process all the ingredients mentioned above in a Juicer or blender, and stir well to combine.

Green with Envy

Serving size: 1 cup (240 ml)

Servings per recipe: Approximately 1

Nutritional Information per serving:

- Calories: 60
- Total fat: 0.4 g
- Saturated fat: 0.1 g
- Trans fat: 0 g
- Cholesterol: 0 mg
- Sodium: 72 mg
- Total carbohydrates: 14 g
- Dietary fiber: 3.4 g
- Sugars: 8 g
- Protein: 2 g

Ingredients

- ¼ cup broccoli florets
- ¼ cup cucumber
- ¼ cup kale leaves
- ¼ cup green bell peppers
- ½ cup tomatoes
- ½ cup celery

Instructions

1. Process all the ingredients mentioned above in a Juicer or blender, and stir well to combine.

Carrot and cucumber Booster

Serving size: 1 cup (240 ml)

Servings per recipe: Approximately 1

Nutritional Information per serving:

- Calories: 50
- Total fat: 0.3 g
- Saturated fat: 0.1 g
- Trans fat: 0 g
- Cholesterol: 0 mg
- Sodium: 58 mg
- Total carbohydrates: 11 g
- Dietary fiber: 2.8 g
- Sugars: 6.1 g
- Protein: 1.8 g

Ingredients

- ½ cup carrots
- ½ cup cucumber
- ½ cup sweet potatoes
- ½ cup carrot greens
- ¼ cup arugula
- ¼ cup lemongrass

Instructions

1. Process all the ingredients mentioned above in a Juicer or blender, and stir well to combine.

The apple booster

Serving size: 1 cup (240 ml)

Servings per recipe: Approximately 1

Nutritional Information per serving:

- Calories: 120
- Total fat: 0.4 g
- Saturated fat: 0.1 g
- Trans fat: 0 g
- Cholesterol: 0 mg
- Sodium: 8 mg
- Total carbohydrates: 32 g
- Dietary fiber: 3 g
- Sugars: 5 g
- Protein: 1 g

Ingredients

- Two carrots
- One cup of diced red and green apple
- One fresh lemon
- One half-inch block of Ginger
- Put all the ingredients through a blender and serve fresh.

Instructions

1. Mix everything in a Juicer or blender and drink fresh.

This tasty recipe for diabetic juice has a very healthy base that not only lowers the chance of developing diabetes and keeps sugar levels in check but also has many other positive effects on one's health.

The Greenland drink

Serving size: 1 cup (240 ml)

Servings per recipe: Approximately 1

Nutritional Information per serving:

- Calories: 68
- Total fat: 0.5 g
- Saturated fat: 0.1 g
- Trans fat: 0 g
- Cholesterol: 0 mg
- Sodium: 126 mg
- Total carbohydrates: 17 g
- Dietary fiber: 3.5 g
- Sugars: 10.2 g
- Protein: 3.1 g

Ingredients

- One bunch of chard

- Half a bunch of kale

- One small green cabbage

- One green apple

- Two celery ribs

- One lemon

Instructions

1. Everything should be juiced up beautifully, and the drink should be served immediately.

Because it contains the goodness of all the major green vegetables, which are both powerful detoxifiers and promote digestion, this is undoubtedly one of the greatest juicing recipes for those with diabetes.

The veggie land drink

Serving size: 1 cup (240 ml)

Servings per recipe: Approximately 1

Nutritional Information per serving:

- Calories: 63
- Total Fat: 0.6 g
- Saturated Fat: 0.1 g
- Trans Fat: 0 g
- Cholesterol: 0 mg
- Sodium: 183 mg
- Total Carbohydrate: 15 g
- Dietary Fiber: 4.2 g
- Sugars: 8.3 g
- Protein: 3.1 g

Ingredients

- One-and-a-half Beet
- Four carrots
- Two tomatoes
- One clove of garlic cloves
- One bunch of spinach
- Five romaine leaves
- Some parsley leaves
- Two celery ribs
- Some watercress
- Salt as per taste

Instructions

1. The ingredients should be juiced well, and the salt should be mixed in at the end.

2. It is now time to serve the beverage.

Once you notice the positive effects juicing has on your health, this is one of the amazing recipes for diabetics that you will get obsessed with.

The bitter melon juice

Serving size: 1 cup (240 ml)

Servings per recipe: Approximately 1

Nutritional Information per serving:

- Calories: 75 kcal
- Total Fat: 0 g
- Saturated Fat: 0 g
- Trans Fat: 0 g
- Cholesterol: 0 mg
- Sodium: 10 mg
- Total Carbohydrates: 19 g
- Dietary Fiber: 1 g
- Sugars: 6 g
- Protein: 1 g

Ingredients

- Two bitter melons
- Some water

Instructions

1.   Fresh consumption can be achieved via juicing, blending, or both, depending on your preference. You may also make the melons taste better by juicing them with cucumber, green apples, or lemons. This is an alternative method.

One could call this the "wonder fruit" for its effectiveness in lowering high blood glucose levels. You can add some additional fruits to the juice if the flavor of the original fruit is not to your liking.

The sweet potato juice

Serving size: 1 cup (240 ml)

Servings per recipe: Approximately 1

Nutritional Information per serving:

- Calories: 120 kcal
- Total Fat: 0.5 g
- Saturated Fat: 0 g
- Trans Fat: 0 g
- Cholesterol: 0 mg
- Sodium: 55 mg
- Total Carbohydrates: 28 g
- Dietary Fiber: 3 g
- Sugars: 15 g
- Protein: 2 g

Ingredients

- One sweet potato
- One green apple
- Two celery ribs
- One one-inch block of Ginger
- Some cinnamon powder

Instructions

1. All ingredients should be juiced, and the drink should be served immediately.

Because it is high in fiber and does a wonderful job of helping to maintain the glucose level in the blood, this is another excellent option on the list of diabetic juicing recipes.

The broccoli juice

Serving size: 1 cup (240 ml)

Servings per recipe: Approximately 1

Nutritional Information per serving:

- Calories: 50 kcal
- Total Fat: 0.5 g
- Saturated Fat: 0 g
- Trans Fat: 0 g
- Cholesterol: 0 mg
- Sodium: 170 mg
- Total Carbohydrates: 10 g
- Dietary Fiber: 3 g
- Sugars: 4 g
- Protein: 4 g

Ingredients

- One broccoli head

- Two carrots as per the taste preference

- Two apples

Instructions

1.   Blend these ingredients and serve the drink fresh.

2.   If you have type 2 diabetes, this is the perfect drink to supply Sulforaphane to the body for controlling glucose-producing enzymes.

The tomato cleanser drink

Serving size: 1 cup (240 ml)

Servings per recipe: Approximately 1

Nutritional Information per serving:

- Calories: 60 kcal
- Total Fat: 0.5 g
- Saturated Fat: 0 g
- Trans Fat: 0 g
- Cholesterol: 0 mg
- Sodium: 400 mg
- Total Carbohydrates: 12 g
- Dietary Fiber: 2 g
- Sugars: 7 g
- Protein: 2 g

Ingredients

- Four big tomatoes, de-seeded

- A bunch of lettuce

Instructions

1. These two should be juiced, and the drink should be served immediately.

This beverage has a substantial amount of the beneficial vitamins and minerals found in tomatoes, and it plays a vital role in assisting with maintaining healthy cardiac function.

The pepper magic drink

Serving size: 1 cup (240 ml)

Servings per recipe: Approximately 1

Nutritional Information per serving:

- Calories: 70 kcal
- Total Fat: 0.5 g
- Saturated Fat: 0 g
- Trans Fat: 0 g
- Cholesterol: 0 mg
- Sodium: 10 mg
- Total Carbohydrates: 16 g
- Dietary Fiber: 2 g
- Sugars: 11 g
- Protein: 2 g

Ingredients

- One bunch of spinach leaves

- One red bell pepper or capsicum

- Two celery sticks

- One kiwi

Instructions

1. Blend everything just fine, and the drink is ready.

Antioxidants are very good at controlling sugar levels in the blood as they flush out toxins. This drink has plenty of antioxidants like lycopene.

The dandelion diabetic concoction

Serving size: 1 cup (240 ml)

Servings per recipe: Approximately 1

Nutritional Information per serving:

- Calories: 70 kcal
- Total Fat: 0 g
- Saturated Fat: 0 g
- Trans Fat: 0 g
- Cholesterol: 0 mg
- Sodium: 10 mg
- Total Carbohydrates: 18 g
- Dietary Fiber: 4 g
- Sugars: 11 g
- Protein: 2 g

Ingredients

- One big bunch of dandelion leaves

- Ten celery ribs

- Four green apples

- One lemon

Instructions

1. Finely juice everything, and serve the drink as soon as it is made.

Reducing inflammation and lowering blood glucose levels are two of the many benefits that type 2 diabetics who use this recipe for diabetic juicing can expect to experience.

Carrot-Apple-Ginger Juice

Serving size: 1 cup (240 ml)

Servings per recipe: Approximately 1

Nutritional Information per serving:

- Calories: 120 kcal
- Total Fat: 0.5 g
- Saturated Fat: 0 g
- Trans Fat: 0 g
- Cholesterol: 0 mg
- Sodium: 60 mg
- Total Carbohydrates: 30 g
- Dietary Fiber: 4 g
- Sugars: 2 g
- Protein: 2 g

Ingredients

- Six ½ carrots

- ½ apple

- ½ apple

- 1/5 lemon

- 1 1/3 inch ginger

Instructions

1.   Wash all the ingredients.

2.   After cutting the lemon in quarters with the skin still attached, put the lemon directly into the press. Without a juice press, peel the lemon and squeeze the juice into the bowl with the other ingredients.

3.   Grind the remaining ingredients and press them together.

Cucumber tomato Booster

Serving size: 1 cup (240 ml)

Servings per recipe: Approximately 1

Nutritional Information per serving:

- Calories: 50 kcal
- Total Fat: 0.5 g
- Saturated Fat: 0 g
- Trans Fat: 0 g
- Cholesterol: 0 mg
- Sodium: 10 mg
- Total Carbohydrates: 12 g
- Dietary Fiber: 3 g
- Sugars: 7 g
- Protein: 2 g

Ingredients

- One sliced Cucumber

- One Tomato

- Coriander leaves

Instructions

1. Take a blender jar. Put sliced cucumber and tomato pieces.

2. Add Coriander leaves to the blender jar.

3. Add one glass of water.

4. Blend the juice. Pour in a glass to serve.

5. The Cucumber-tomato-Coriander juice is ready. Drink this juice to beat the heat and reverse diabetes.

Cucumber-Lemon-Ginger-juice recipe for diabetics

Serving size: 1 cup (240 ml)

Servings per recipe: Approximately 1

Nutritional Information per serving:

- Calories: 70 kcal
- Total Fat: 0.5 g
- Saturated Fat: 0 g
- Trans Fat: 0 g
- Cholesterol: 0 mg
- Sodium: 20 mg
- Total Carbohydrates: 17 g
- Dietary Fiber: 2 g
- Sugars: 7 g
- Protein: 1 g

Ingredients

- One sliced Cucumber
- One sliced Ginger
- One lemon
- Coriander leaves

Instructions

1. Add sliced cucumber and ginger pieces and coriander leaves in a Juicer or blender jar.

2. In a Juicer or blender, combine one glass of water with the juice of half a lemon.

3. Combine the ingredients very thoroughly. When you're ready to serve it, pour it into a glass.

Cucumber, ginger, lemon, and coriander juice are now ready to be consumed. Consume it every week and track its effects on your blood sugar levels.

Serving size: 1 cup (240 ml)

Servings per recipe: Approximately 1

Nutritional Information per serving:

- Calories: 40 kcal
- Total Fat: 0.5 g
- Saturated Fat: 0 g
- Trans Fat: 0 g
- Cholesterol: 0 mg
- Sodium: 20 mg
- Total Carbohydrates: 8 g
- Dietary Fiber: 2 g
- Sugars: 2 g
- Protein: 2 g

Ingredients

- One sliced Cucumber

- One Bitter gourd

- One green apple

- Two tablespoons of Chia seeds

Instructions

1.   Add sliced cucumber, green apple, and bitter gourd pieces in a Juicer or blender jar.

2.   Add a glass of water and two tablespoons of chia seeds.

3.   Blend this well and pour it into a glass.

4.   The Cucumber-Bitter gourd-Green apple-Chia seeds juice is ready. Regular consumption of this will help in the reduction of blood sugar levels.

Delicious Tomato juice for diabetics

Serving size: 1 cup (240 ml)

Servings per recipe: Approximately 1

Nutritional Information per serving:

- Calories: 50 kcal
- Total Fat: 0.5 g
- Saturated Fat: 0 g
- Trans Fat: 0 g
- Cholesterol: 0 mg
- Sodium: 30 mg
- Total Carbohydrates: 10 g
- Dietary Fiber: 2 g
- Sugars: 6 g
- Protein: 2 g

Ingredient

- Tomato is the only ingredient required for this juice recipe.

Instructions

1. Cut fresh Tomato into pieces.

2. Add them to a blender jar and add one glass of water.

3. Blend them and pour them into a glass to serve.

4. The tomato juice is ready. It can be consumed every day to see visible results.

Bitter melon and apple juice for diabetes

Serving size: 1 cup (240 ml)

Servings per recipe: Approximately 1

Nutritional Information per serving:

- Calories: 80 kcal
- Total Fat: 0.5 g
- Saturated Fat: 0 g
- Trans Fat: 0 g
- Cholesterol: 0 mg
- Sodium: 10 mg
- Total Carbohydrates: 20 g
- Dietary Fiber: 4 g
- Sugars: 4 g
- Protein: 2 g

Ingredients

- One bitter melon
- ½ cup of water
- One small apple
- Half a lemon
- Pinch of salt

Instructions

1. Blend everything and drink fresh.

2. You can toss in cucumber and Ginger too. Do not add too much apple as it will increase your blood sugar. Adjust the ingredients to your needs.

Carrot and apple juice for sugar patients

Serving size: 1 cup (240 ml)

Servings per recipe: Approximately 1

Nutritional Information per serving:

- Calories: 90 kcal
- Total Fat: 0.5 g
- Saturated Fat: 0 g
- Trans Fat: 0 g
- Cholesterol: 0 mg
- Sodium: 60 mg
- Total Carbohydrates: 22 g
- Dietary Fiber: 4 g
- Sugars: 6 g
- Protein: 2 g

Ingredients

- One carrot

- ½ cup of green and red apple combination

- Ginger and lemon

Instructions

1. Blend everything in a Juicer or blender and drink fresh.

This is one of the healthiest drinks to add to your favorite juices. It is a rich source of nutrients, like vitamins and minerals. It is mild in its taste and has a tinge of sweetness.

A mix of green and sweet juicing recipes for diabetics

Serving size: 1 cup (240 ml)

Servings per recipe: Approximately 1

Nutritional Information per serving:

- Calories: 90 kcal
- Total Fat: 0.5 g
- Saturated Fat: 0 g
- Trans Fat: 0 g
- Cholesterol: 0 mg
- Sodium: 60 mg
- Total Carbohydrates: 22 g
- Dietary Fiber: 4 g
- Sugars: 4 g
- Protein: 2 g

Ingredients

- One cucumber
- One green apple
- One carrot
- One cup of celery and spinach
- Ginger and lemon

Instructions

1. Blend everything and drink fresh.

Cucumbers are a delicious way to dilute the juices and mask their taste. Also, you can toss Ginger and lemon in your juicing recipes that are for diabetics. It makes everything a bit more pleasant for your taste buds!

Green Goodness

Serving size: 1 cup (240 ml)

Servings per recipe: Approximately 1

Nutritional Information per serving:

- Calories: 110 kcal
- Total Fat: 0.5 g
- Saturated Fat: 0 g
- Trans Fat: 0 g
- Cholesterol: 0 mg
- Sodium: 70 mg
- Total Carbohydrates: 27 g
- Dietary Fiber: 3 g
- Sugars: 7 g
- Protein: 3 g

Ingredients:

- 2 cups fresh kale leaves
- 2 cups of fresh spinach leaves
- 1 cup mixed berries (such as strawberries, blueberries, and raspberries)
- 1 cup fresh almond milk
- One tbsp. of vanilla protein powder
- 1 tbsp. chia seeds

Instructions:

1. Wash and chop the kale and spinach leaves.

2. Combine the kale, spinach, mixed red berries, fresh almond milk, delicious vanilla protein powder, and chia seeds in a Juicer or blender.

3. Blend until mixed well and creamy.

4. Pour the juice into a glass and serve immediately.

This Green Goodness Juice is a delicious and nutritious way to start your day, providing essential vitamins and minerals, healthy fats, and plant-based protein to support overall health and manage diabetes. The kale and spinach provide antioxidants, fiber, and anti-inflammatory, while the mixed berries add natural sweetness and boost vitamins. The almond milk and protein powder help to increase the protein content of the juice, making it a more filling and satisfying drink, while the chia seeds add healthy fats and fiber. This juice is a perfect way to start your day or enjoy it as a snack anytime.

Acai Bowl: acai berry puree, mixed red berries, fresh almond milk, delicious vanilla protein powder, rolled oats

Serving size: 1 cup (240 ml)

Servings per recipe: Approximately 1

Nutritional Information per serving:

- Calories: 360 kcal
- Total Fat: 10 g
- Saturated Fat: 1 g
- Trans Fat: 0 g
- Cholesterol: 0 mg
- Sodium: 120 mg
- Total Carbohydrates: 50 g
- Dietary Fiber: 11 g
- Sugars: 4 g
- Protein: 22 g

Ingredients:

- One pack of frozen acai berry puree

- One cup of fresh mixed berries

- One cup of fresh almond milk

- One small scoop of vanilla protein powder

- 1/4 cup rolled oats

Instructions:

1. Defrost the acai berry puree according to package instructions.

2. Combine the acai berry puree, mixed red berries, fresh almond milk, delicious vanilla protein powder, and rolled oats in a Juicer or blender.

3. Blend until mixed well and creamy.

4. Pour the juice into a small bowl and top with additional mixed berries, rolled oats, and other toppings of your choice (such as sliced almonds, chia seeds, or fresh fruit).

5. Serve immediately and enjoy!

This Acai Bowl is a delicious and nutritious way to start your day, providing essential vitamins and minerals, healthy fats, and plant-based protein to support overall health and manage diabetes. The acai berry puree is a great source of antioxidants and fiber, while the mixed berries add natural sweetness and a boost of vitamins. The almond milk and protein powder help to increase the protein content of the bowl, making it a more filling and satisfying meal. At the same time, rolled oats provide fiber and a slower release of carbohydrates to help regulate blood sugar levels. This bowl is a perfect way to start your day or enjoy it as a snack anytime.

Raspberry Ripple: raspberries, banana, fresh almond milk, delicious vanilla protein powder, rolled oats

Serving size: 1 cup (240 ml)

Servings per recipe: Approximately 1

Nutritional Information per serving:

- Calories: 300 kcal
- Total Fat: 6 g
- Saturated Fat: 0.5 g
- Trans Fat: 0 g
- Cholesterol: 0 mg
- Sodium: 120 mg
- Total Carbohydrates: 46 g
- Dietary Fiber: 11 g
- Sugars: 2 g
- Protein: 18 g

Ingredients:

- One cup raspberries
- 1/4 banana
- One cup of fresh almond milk
- One tbsp. of vanilla protein powder
- 1/4 cup rolled oats

Instructions:

1. Combine the raspberries, banana, fresh almond milk, delicious vanilla protein powder, and rolled oats in a Juicer or blender.

2. Blend until mixed well and creamy.

3. Pour the juice into a glass and serve immediately.

This Raspberry Ripple Juice is a delicious and nutritious way to start your day, providing essential vitamins and minerals, healthy fats, and plant-based protein to support overall health and manage diabetes. The raspberries add a sweet and tart flavor, while the banana provides natural sweetness and creaminess. The almond milk and protein powder help to increase the protein content of the juice, making it a more filling and satisfying drink. At the same time, rolled oats provide fiber and a slower release of carbohydrates to help regulate blood sugar levels. This juice is a perfect way to start your day or enjoy it as a snack anytime.

Blueberry Blast: blueberries, banana, fresh almond milk, delicious vanilla protein powder, rolled oats

Serving size: 1 cup (240 ml)

Servings per recipe: Approximately 1

Nutritional Information per serving:

- Calories: 320 kcal
- Total Fat: 6 g
- Saturated Fat: 0.5 g
- Trans Fat: 0 g
- Cholesterol: 0 mg
- Sodium: 120 mg
- Total Carbohydrates: 48 g
- Dietary Fiber: 10 g
- Sugars: 2 g

Ingredients:

- One cup blueberries

- One banana

- One cup of fresh almond milk

- One tbsp. vanilla protein powder

- 1/4 cup rolled oats

Instructions:

1. Combine the blueberries, banana, fresh almond milk, delicious vanilla protein powder, and rolled oats in a Juicer or blender.

2. Blend until mixed well and creamy.

3. Pour the juice into a glass and serve immediately.

This Blueberry Blast Juice is a delicious and nutritious way to start your day, providing essential vitamins and minerals, healthy fats, and plant-based protein to support overall health and manage diabetes. The blueberries add a sweet and fruity flavor, while the banana provides natural sweetness and creaminess. The almond milk and protein powder help to increase the protein content of the juice, making it a more filling and satisfying drink. At the same time, rolled oats provide fiber and a slower release of carbohydrates to help regulate blood sugar levels. This juice is a perfect way to start your day or enjoy it as a snack anytime.

Cherry Almond: cherries, almond milk butter, vanilla powder, rolled oats

Serving size: 1 cup (240 ml)

Servings per recipe: Approximately 1

Nutritional Information per serving:

- Calories: 350 kcal
- Total Fat: 10 g
- Saturated Fat: 1 g
- Trans Fat: 0 g
- Cholesterol: 0 mg
- Sodium: 120 mg
- Total Carbohydrates: 57 g
- Dietary Fiber: 11 g
- Sugars: 5 g
- Protein: 15 g

Ingredients:

- One cup of cherries (fresh or frozen)
- One cup of fresh almond milk
- One tablespoon of almond butter
- One tbsp. of vanilla protein powder
- 1/4 cup rolled oats

Instructions:

1.   In a Juicer or blender, combine the cherries, almond milk, butter, vanilla protein powder, and rolled oats.

2.   Blend until mixed well and creamy.

3.   Pour the juice into a glass and serve immediately.

This Cherry Almond Juice is a delicious and nutritious way to start your day, providing essential vitamins and minerals, healthy fats, and plant-based protein to support overall health and manage diabetes. The cherries add a sweet and tart flavor, while the almond milk and butter provide healthy fats and natural sweetness. The vanilla protein powder helps increase the juice's protein content, making it a more filling and satisfying drink. At the same time, rolled oats provide fiber and a slower release of carbohydrates to help regulate blood sugar levels. This juice is a perfect way to start your day or enjoy it as a snack anytime.

Vanilla Bean: vanilla almond milk, fresh banana, delicious protein powder, rolled oats, vanilla extract.

Serving size: 1 cup (240 ml)

Servings per recipe: Approximately 1

Nutritional Information per serving:

- Calories: 380 kcal
- Total Fat: 9 g
- Saturated Fat: 1 g
- Trans Fat: 0 g
- Cholesterol: 0 mg
- Sodium: 210 mg
- Total Carbohydrates: 59 g
- Dietary Fiber: 11 g
- Sugars: 9 g
- Protein: 19 g

Ingredients:

- One cup of delicious vanilla almond milk

- One fresh banana

- One tbsp. of vanilla protein powder

- 1/4 cup rolled oats

- One teaspoon of vanilla extract

Instructions:

1. Combine the vanilla almond milk, banana, vanilla protein powder, oats, and vanilla extract in a Juicer or blender.

2. Blend until mixed well and creamy.

3. Pour the juice into a glass and serve immediately.

This Vanilla Bean Juice is a delicious and nutritious way to start your day, providing essential vitamins and minerals, healthy fats, and plant-based protein to support overall health and manage diabetes. The vanilla almond milk and extract provide a sweet and creamy flavor, while the banana provides natural sweetness. The vanilla protein powder helps increase the juice's protein content, making it a more filling and satisfying drink. At the same time, rolled oats provide fiber and a slower release of carbohydrates to help regulate blood sugar levels. This juice is a perfect way to start your day or enjoy it as a snack anytime.

Banana Oat: banana, fresh almond milk, delicious vanilla protein powder, rolled oats, cinnamon

Serving size: 1 cup (240 ml)

Servings per recipe: Approximately 1

Nutritional Information per serving:

- Calories: 375 kcal
- Total Fat: 7 g
- Saturated Fat: 1 g
- Trans Fat: 0 g
- Cholesterol: 0 mg
- Sodium: 230 mg
- Total Carbohydrates: 60 g
- Dietary Fiber: 9 g
- Sugars: 5 g
- Protein: 20 g

Ingredients:

- One banana
- One cup of fresh almond milk
- One tbsp. of vanilla protein powder
- 1/4 cup rolled oats
- One teaspoon of cinnamon

Instructions:

1.   In a Juicer or blender, combine the banana, fresh almond milk, delicious vanilla protein powder, rolled oats, and cinnamon.

2.   Blend until mixed well and creamy.

3.   Pour the juice into a glass and serve immediately.

This Banana Oat Juice is a delicious and nutritious way to start your day, providing essential vitamins and minerals, healthy fats, and plant-based protein to support overall health and manage diabetes. The banana provides natural sweetness and creaminess, while the almond milk and vanilla protein powder help increase the juice's protein content, making it a more filling and satisfying drink. The rolled oats and cinnamon provide fiber, flavor, and a slower release of carbohydrates to help regulate blood sugar levels. This juice is a perfect way to start your day or enjoy it as a snack anytime.

Avocado Dream: avocado, mixed red berries, fresh almond milk, delicious vanilla protein powder, chia seeds

Serving size: 1 cup (240 ml)

Servings per recipe: Approximately 1

Nutritional Information per serving:

- Total Fat: 28 g
- Saturated Fat: 3 g
- Trans Fat: 0 g
- Cholesterol: 0 mg
- Sodium: 260 mg
- Total Carbohydrates: 35 g
- Dietary Fiber: 15 g
- Sugars: 11 g
- Protein: 20 g

Ingredients:

- One avocado

- One cup of mixed berries

- One cup of fresh almond milk

- One tbsp. of vanilla protein powder

- One tablespoon of chia seeds

Instructions:

1.   Combine the avocado, mixed red berries, fresh almond milk, delicious vanilla protein powder, and chia seeds in a Juicer or blender.

2.   Blend until mixed well and creamy.

3.   Pour the juice into a glass and serve immediately.

This Avocado Dream Juice is a delicious and nutritious way to start your day, providing essential vitamins and minerals, healthy fats, and plant-based protein to support overall health and manage diabetes. The avocado provides healthy monounsaturated and polyunsaturated fats, while the mixed berries add a sweet and fruity flavor. The almond milk and vanilla protein powder help to increase the protein content of the juice, making it a more filling and satisfying drink. At the same time, the chia seeds provide fiber, essential fatty acids, and a slower release of carbohydrates to help regulate blood sugar levels. This juice is a perfect way to start your day or enjoy it as a snack anytime.

CONCLUSIONS

Juicing can be an excellent way for people with diabetes to manage their health and improve their nutrition. By incorporating a variety of low glycemic index fruits and vegetables into your juicing regimen, you can help regulate blood sugar levels, support overall health, and achieve your health and wellness goals.

However, it is important to note that juicing should be just one part of a well-rounded and balanced diet. Working with a healthcare provider is also important to ensure that your juicing regimen is appropriate for your individual needs and health status.

In this diabetic juicing cookbook, we have provided a range of delicious and nutritious juice recipes to help you start your juicing journey. By incorporating these recipes into your daily routine, you can support your health and well-being and enjoy the benefits of a properly balanced and healthy diet. So get ready to start juicing, and enjoy the delicious and nutritious results!

Printed in Great Britain
by Amazon

22200140R00051